# THE ULTIMATE CKD STAGE 4 COOKBOOK FOR SENIORS

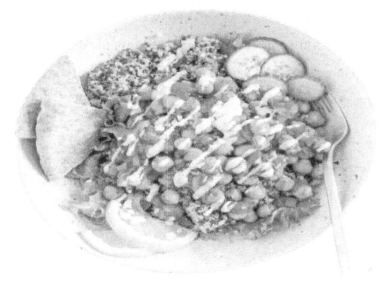

Easy And Delicious Low Sodium, Low Potassium And Low Phosphorus Diet Recipes To Manage Chronic Kidney Disease And Improve Renal Function

Katherine J. Filer

**Copyright 2024, Katherine J. Filer**

All rights reserved. No part of this publication may be reproduced, stored in a retrieval system, or transmitted, in any form or by any means, electronic, mechanical, photocopying, recording, or otherwise, without the prior written permission of the author, except in the case of brief quotations embodied in critical reviews and certain other noncommercial uses permitted by copyright law.

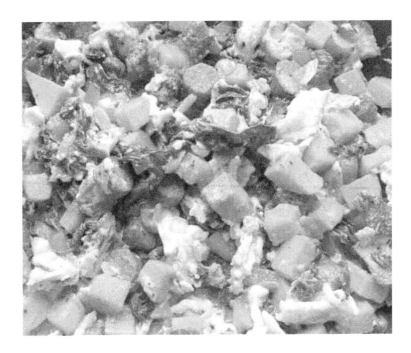

# Table of Contents

# INTRODUCTION

Margaret, a spirited senior who found herself navigating the challenging landscape of Chronic Kidney Disease (CKD) Stage 4. Struggling with managing her diet amidst the complexities of her condition, she embarked on a quest to find a solution that would not only nourish her body but also delight her taste buds. Little did she know that her journey would lead her to the ultimate CKD Stage 4 cookbook, a treasure trove of culinary wonders tailored specifically for seniors like her.

As Margaret flipped through the pages of this cookbook, she discovered a world of tantalizing recipes carefully crafted to cater to her dietary needs. From succulent chicken dishes to vibrant salads brimming with low-potassium fruits and vegetables, every recipe whispered promises of both health and gastronomic pleasure. The cookbook wasn't just a collection of recipes; it was a roadmap to regaining control over her health and savoring life's flavors despite the challenges of CKD Stage 4.

Within those pages, Margaret found more than just meals; she found empowerment. Each recipe came with meticulous guidelines and nutritional insights, guiding her towards optimal choices to support kidney health. From protein-rich options to flavorful yet kidney-friendly seasonings, the cookbook wasn't just about sustenance; it was about reclaiming the joy of eating while managing a chronic condition.

But the real magic lay beyond the ingredients and instructions. It was the transformative power these recipes held, which is the potential to slow disease progression, alleviate symptoms, and infuse vitality into her days. The cookbook wasn't merely a guide; it was a companion in her health journey, offering hope and inspiration with every dish.

Now, as Margaret shared her experiences with newfound energy and enthusiasm, she realized the profound impact this cookbook could have on the lives of others like her. It wasn't just a cookbook; it was a beacon of possibility, a way to savor life's moments and relish the pleasures of food, all while managing CKD Stage 4.

Dear reader, welcome to the ultimate CKD Stage 4 cookbook for seniors, a guide not just to meals, but to a vibrant and fulfilling life even in the face of chronic health challenges. Let its pages be your gateway to a world where health and flavor coexist, where every dish is a step towards wellness and joy. Embrace this journey, and discover the transformative power of food tailored for your well-being.

# CHAPTER 1

## Understanding CKD (Chronic Kidney Disease)

Understanding Chronic Kidney Disease (CKD) Stage 4 involves recognizing a significant decline in kidney function. At this stage, kidneys are moderately to severely impaired, operating at a glomerular filtration rate (GFR) of 15-29 milliliters per minute per 1.73 square meters. CKD Stage 4 is characterized by several distinctive features, including the increased accumulation of waste products and fluids in the body, leading to a higher risk of complications.

Individuals in Stage 4 CKD often experience symptoms such as fatigue, fluid retention causing swelling (edema), changes in urination patterns, increased blood pressure, and anemia due to decreased production of red blood cells by the kidneys. Additionally, electrolyte imbalances like high potassium levels may occur, impacting heart health. Dietary and lifestyle modifications, alongside proper medical management, become crucial at this stage to slow disease progression and manage associated symptoms.

Patients in Stage 4 CKD are usually under the care of nephrologists and healthcare providers. They require regular monitoring of kidney function, blood pressure, and other related health parameters. Treatment goals aim to manage complications, prevent further decline in kidney function, and prepare individuals for potential renal replacement therapy, such as dialysis or kidney transplantation, in advanced stages of CKD. Education, support, and adherence to a kidney-friendly diet and medication regimen play pivotal roles in enhancing quality of life and managing CKD Stage 4 effectively.

# Foods To Eat And Avoid

**Foods to Eat:**

### 1. High-Quality Protein:
- Opt for high-quality protein sources like fish, poultry, egg whites, and small portions of lean meats. These sources contain essential amino acids without excessive phosphorus content.

### 2. Low-Potassium Fruits and Vegetables:
- Consume low-potassium fruits such as apples, berries, and grapes. Opt for vegetables like green beans, cabbage, and onions, which are lower in potassium. Cooking methods like boiling or leaching can help reduce potassium content.

### 3. Low-Phosphorus Foods:
- Choose foods lower in phosphorus like rice, pasta, bread, and certain cereals. Dairy substitutes such as almond milk or rice milk are lower in phosphorus than regular milk.

### 4. Healthy Fats:
- Include heart-healthy fats like olive oil, avocado, and nuts in moderation. These fats provide essential nutrients without impacting kidney health.

### 5. Limited Fluid Intake:
- Monitor fluid intake to prevent fluid buildup. Consume drinks like herbal teas and limit high-sugar beverages or those containing phosphorus additives.

### Foods to Limit or Avoid:

### 1. High-Potassium Foods:
- Limit potassium-rich foods such as bananas, oranges, tomatoes, and potatoes. These foods can elevate potassium levels, posing risks for heart complications.

### 2. High-Phosphorus Foods:
- Avoid or limit phosphorus-rich foods like dairy products, processed foods, nuts, seeds, and colas. High phosphorus levels can negatively impact bone health.

### 3. Excessive Sodium:

- Reduce sodium intake by avoiding processed foods, canned soups, and packaged snacks. High sodium can elevate blood pressure and cause fluid retention.

### 4. High-Protein Foods:

- Limit intake of high-protein foods like red meat, which can burden the kidneys with excess waste products.

### 5. Fluid Intake Control:

- Monitor and restrict fluid intake to avoid fluid overload, which can lead to swelling, high blood pressure, and heart strain.

# Core Benefits of following a CKD Diet

### 1. Slows Disease Progression:

A CKD Stage 4 diet helps slow the progression of kidney damage in seniors. By controlling intake of certain nutrients like protein, phosphorus, potassium, and sodium, the diet reduces stress on the kidneys, potentially preserving remaining kidney function.

### 2. Manages Symptoms and Complications:

This diet helps manage and alleviate symptoms commonly associated with CKD Stage 4 in seniors. By regulating fluid intake, it minimizes complications such as fluid retention, swelling (edema), and high blood pressure, improving overall comfort and reducing the risk of cardiovascular issues.

### 3. Optimizes Nutrition:
Tailoring the diet ensures seniors receive adequate and balanced nutrition. Despite restrictions, a CKD Stage 4 diet allows for the inclusion of essential nutrients through carefully chosen foods, contributing to overall health and well-being in older adults.

### 4. Reduces Risk of Malnutrition:
Seniors with CKD Stage 4 face a higher risk of malnutrition due to dietary limitations. A well-structured diet plan, often devised with the guidance of a dietitian, helps seniors maintain adequate nourishment by selecting foods that are both kidney-friendly and nutrient-dense.

### 5. Preserves Bone Health:
By moderating phosphorus intake, this diet supports bone health in seniors. High phosphorus levels can lead to bone problems, and the CKD Stage 4 diet focuses on reducing phosphorus-rich foods to maintain optimal bone strength.

### 6. Manages Medication and Treatment Effects:
Certain medications and treatments for CKD can impact appetite, digestion, and nutrient absorption in seniors.

Following a specialized diet helps counteract these effects and supports the effectiveness of prescribed treatments.

### 7. Improves Quality of Life:
By providing a structured and manageable eating plan, a CKD Stage 4 diet contributes to a better quality of life for seniors. It empowers them with the knowledge and tools to take an active role in managing their health, reducing stress associated with dietary uncertainties.

### 8. Promotes Cardiovascular Health:
Controlling sodium intake helps manage blood pressure and fluid retention, supporting heart health in seniors with CKD Stage 4. By minimizing strain on the cardiovascular system, the diet reduces the risk of heart-related complications.

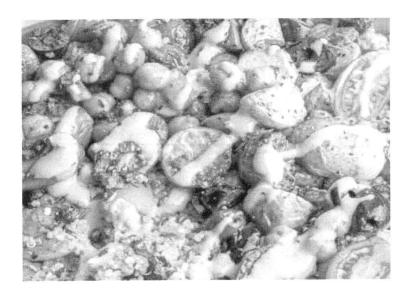

# 20 healthy shopping ingredients suitable for a CKD Stage 4 diet:

## Protein Sources:

1. Skinless Poultry: Chicken and turkey are lean protein sources with lower phosphorus content.
2. Fish: Select varieties like salmon, tuna, and trout which are high in omega-3 fatty acids and lower in phosphorus.
3. Egg Whites: Rich in high-quality protein and low in phosphorus, egg whites are an excellent option.

## Fruits:

4. Apples: Low in potassium, apples are a kidney-friendly fruit choice.
5. Berries: Blueberries, strawberries, and raspberries are lower-potassium fruit options packed with antioxidants.
6. Grapes: Red and green grapes are low in potassium and can be a tasty addition.

## Vegetables:

7. Green Beans: A low-potassium vegetable rich in nutrients and fiber.
8. Cabbage: Low in potassium and versatile for cooking or salads.
9. Onions: Add flavor to dishes without adding significant potassium.

### Grains:

10. White Rice: A lower-phosphorus alternative to whole grains.

11. Pasta: Choose pasta made from refined grains for lower phosphorus content.

12. Bread: Look for white or refined bread for lower phosphorus and potassium levels.

### Dairy Substitutes:

13. Almond Milk: Low in phosphorus and potassium compared to regular dairy milk.

14. Rice Milk: Another dairy substitute with lower phosphorus content.

### Healthy Fats:

15. Olive Oil: A heart-healthy fat suitable for cooking and dressing.

16. Avocados: Provide healthy fats and are lower in potassium compared to other fruits.

### Beverages:

17. Herbal Teas: Non-caffeinated herbal teas are suitable for fluid intake control.

18. Cranberry Juice (Unsweetened): Lower in potassium compared to some other fruit juices.

### Snack Options:

19. Popcorn: A low-phosphorus and low-potassium snack when prepared without added salt.

20. Rice Cakes: A low-phosphorus, low-potassium option for a snack or light meal.

# Complications of CKD Stage 4 if the right diet isn't adopted

### 1. Progression of Kidney Damage:
Inadequate dietary management can accelerate the progression of kidney damage. Excessive intake of certain nutrients like protein, phosphorus, potassium, and sodium can further burden the kidneys, leading to faster decline in kidney function.

### 2. Fluid Retention and Edema:
Failure to control fluid intake can result in fluid retention and edema (swelling) in various parts of the body, including the legs, ankles, and around the eyes. This can exacerbate high blood pressure and strain the heart.

### 3. Electrolyte Imbalances:
Imbalances in electrolytes like potassium, sodium, and phosphorus can occur, leading to complications such as irregular heartbeats, muscle weakness, and bone problems. Elevated potassium levels (hyperkalemia) pose a significant risk for heart-related issues.

### 4. Cardiovascular Complications:

CKD Stage 4 individuals have a higher risk of cardiovascular diseases. Without proper dietary management, complications like hypertension, fluid overload, and electrolyte imbalances can contribute to an increased risk of heart attacks, strokes, and heart failure.

**5. Bone and Mineral Disorders:**
Inadequate control of phosphorus levels can lead to bone and mineral disorders such as bone pain, weakened bones (renal osteodystrophy), and increased fracture risk.

**6. Malnutrition and Worsened Symptoms:**
Improper nutrition can lead to malnutrition due to restricted food choices and limited nutrient intake. This can further weaken the body, worsen symptoms, and reduce quality of life.

**7. Increased Risk of Hospitalization and Mortality:**
Complications arising from uncontrolled CKD Stage 4 can lead to frequent hospitalizations and an increased risk of mortality. Cardiovascular events and infections become more prevalent without proper dietary and medical management.

**8. Reduced Effectiveness of Treatment:**
Failure to adhere to a suitable diet can diminish the effectiveness of medications and treatments prescribed to manage CKD-related complications. This can result in less effective control of symptoms and disease progression.

# CHAPTER 2

## 30 DAYS MEAL PLAN

**Day 1:**
- Breakfast: Quinoa Breakfast Bowl
- Lunch: Grilled Lemon Herb Chicken
- Dinner: Baked Lemon Herb Salmon
- Snack: Baked Zucchini Chips

**Day 2:**
- Breakfast: Egg White Veggie Omelette
- Lunch: Salmon and Quinoa Salad
- Dinner: Turkey Chili
- Snack: Hummus with Veggie Sticks

**Day 3:**
- Breakfast: Cottage Cheese Pancakes
- Lunch: Vegetable Stir-Fry with Tofu
- Dinner: Baked Herb Chicken with Roasted Vegetables
- Snack: Cottage Cheese and Berry Parfait

**Day 4:**
- Breakfast: Chia Seed Pudding
- Lunch: Turkey and Veggie Lettuce Wraps
- Dinner: Mediterranean Chickpea Salad
- Snack: Baked Sweet Potato Fries

**Day 5:**
- Breakfast: Greek Yogurt Parfait
- Lunch: Lemon Herb Baked Cod
- Dinner: Quinoa and Vegetable Stir-Fry
- Snack: Egg Salad Lettuce Wraps

**Day 6:**
- Breakfast: Sweet Potato Breakfast Hash
- Lunch: Tuna Salad Lettuce Wraps
- Dinner: Herb-Roasted Vegetables
- Snack: Cottage Cheese and Berry Parfait

**Day 7:**
- Breakfast: Rice Cake with Avocado and Tomato
- Lunch: Chicken and Vegetable Skewers
- Dinner: Lemon Garlic Shrimp Pasta
- Snack: Hummus with Veggie Sticks

**Day 8:**
- Breakfast: Coconut Chia Seed Pudding
- Lunch: Vegetable Stir-Fry with Tofu
- Dinner: Baked Herb Chicken with Roasted Vegetables
- Snack: Cottage Cheese and Berry Parfait

**Day 9:**
- Breakfast: Oatmeal with Almond Butter and Banana
- Lunch: Grilled Lemon Herb Chicken
- Dinner: Turkey Chili
- Snack: Baked Zucchini Chips

**Day 10:**
- Breakfast: Egg White Veggie Omelette
- Lunch: Salmon and Quinoa Salad
- Dinner: Baked Lemon Herb Salmon
- Snack: Hummus with Veggie Sticks

**Day 11:**
- Breakfast: Millet Porridge
- Lunch: Vegetable Lentil Soup
- Dinner: Lemon Herb Baked Cod
- Snack: Baked Sweet Potato Fries

**Day 12:**
- Breakfast: Greek Yogurt Parfait
- Lunch: Chicken and Vegetable Skewers
- Dinner: Quinoa and Vegetable Stir-Fry
- Snack: Egg Salad Lettuce Wraps

**Day 13:**
- Breakfast: Sweet Potato Breakfast Hash
- Lunch: Tuna Salad Lettuce Wraps
- Dinner: Mediterranean Chickpea Salad
- Snack: Cottage Cheese and Berry Parfait

**Day 14:**
- Breakfast: Rice Cake with Avocado and Tomato
- Lunch: Lemon Herb Baked Cod
- Dinner: Baked Lemon Herb Salmon
- Snack: Hummus with Veggie Sticks

**Day 15:**
- Breakfast: Chia Seed Pudding
- Lunch: Grilled Lemon Herb Chicken
- Dinner: Baked Lemon Herb Salmon
- Snack: Baked Zucchini Chips

**Day 16:**
- Breakfast: Egg White Veggie Omelette
- Lunch: Salmon and Quinoa Salad
- Dinner: Turkey Chili
- Snack: Hummus with Veggie Sticks

**Day 17:**
- Breakfast: Cottage Cheese Pancakes
- Lunch: Vegetable Stir-Fry with Tofu
- Dinner: Baked Herb Chicken with Roasted Vegetables
- Snack: Cottage Cheese and Berry Parfait

**Day 18:**
- Breakfast: Coconut Chia Seed Pudding
- Lunch: Turkey and Veggie Lettuce Wraps
- Dinner: Mediterranean Chickpea Salad
- Snack: Baked Sweet Potato Fries

**Day 19:**
- Breakfast: Greek Yogurt Parfait
- Lunch: Lemon Herb Baked Cod
- Dinner: Quinoa and Vegetable Stir-Fry
- Snack: Egg Salad Lettuce Wraps

**Day 20:**
- Breakfast: Sweet Potato Breakfast Hash
- Lunch: Tuna Salad Lettuce Wraps
- Dinner: Herb-Roasted Vegetables
- Snack: Cottage Cheese and Berry Parfait

**Day 21:**
- Breakfast: Rice Cake with Avocado and Tomato
- Lunch: Chicken and Vegetable Skewers
- Dinner: Lemon Garlic Shrimp Pasta
- Snack: Hummus with Veggie Sticks

**Day 22:**
- Breakfast: Millet Porridge
- Lunch: Grilled Lemon Herb Chicken
- Dinner: Baked Lemon Herb Salmon
- Snack: Baked Zucchini Chips

**Day 23:**
- Breakfast: Egg White Veggie Omelette
- Lunch: Salmon and Quinoa Salad
- Dinner: Turkey Chili
- Snack: Hummus with Veggie Sticks

**Day 24:**
- Breakfast: Coconut Chia Seed Pudding
- Lunch: Vegetable Stir-Fry with Tofu
- Dinner: Baked Herb Chicken with Roasted Vegetables
- Snack: Cottage Cheese and Berry Parfait

**Day 25:**
- Breakfast: Greek Yogurt Parfait
- Lunch: Lemon Herb Baked Cod
- Dinner: Quinoa and Vegetable Stir-Fry
- Snack: Egg Salad Lettuce Wraps

**Day 26:**
- Breakfast: Sweet Potato Breakfast Hash
- Lunch: Tuna Salad Lettuce Wraps
- Dinner: Herb-Roasted Vegetables
- Snack: Cottage Cheese and Berry Parfait

**Day 27:**
- Breakfast: Rice Cake with Avocado and Tomato
- Lunch: Chicken and Vegetable Skewers
- Dinner: Lemon Garlic Shrimp Pasta
- Snack: Hummus with Veggie Sticks

**Day 28:**
- Breakfast: Millet Porridge
- Lunch: Grilled Lemon Herb Chicken
- Dinner: Baked Lemon Herb Salmon
- Snack: Baked Zucchini Chips

**Day 29:**
- Breakfast: Egg White Veggie Omelette
- Lunch: Salmon and Quinoa Salad
- Dinner: Turkey Chili
- Snack: Hummus with Veggie Sticks

**Day 30:**
- Breakfast: Quinoa Breakfast Bowl
- Lunch: Grilled Lemon Herb Chicken
- Dinner: Baked Lemon Herb Salmon
- Snack: Baked Zucchini Chips

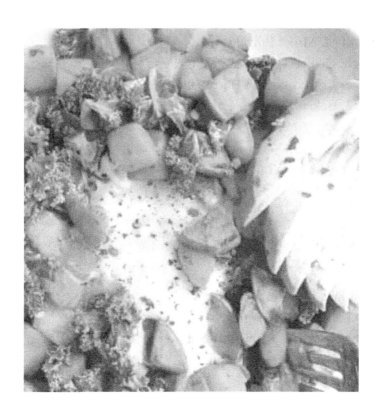

# CHAPTER 3

# CKD Stage 4 Recipes

## BREAKFAST RECIPES

## 1. Quinoa Breakfast Bowl

**Ingredients:**
- 1/2 cup quinoa
- 1 cup water
- 1/4 cup diced strawberries
- 1/4 cup blueberries
- 1 tablespoon chopped almonds
- 1 teaspoon honey (optional)

**Preparation:**
1. Rinse quinoa thoroughly. Cook quinoa with water in a saucepan according to package instructions.
2. Once cooked, place quinoa in a bowl. Top with strawberries, blueberries, chopped almonds, and a drizzle of honey if desired.

**Nutritional Value:**
- Quinoa provides protein and fiber.
- Berries offer antioxidants and vitamins.

- Almonds add healthy fats and a crunch.

**Cooking Time:** Around 15-20 minutes.

# 2. Egg White Veggie Omelette

**Ingredients:**
- 3 egg whites
- 1/4 cup chopped bell peppers
- 1/4 cup chopped spinach
- 1 tablespoon chopped onion
- 1 teaspoon olive oil
- Salt and pepper to taste

**Preparation:**
1. In a bowl, whisk egg whites until frothy. Add salt and pepper.
2. Heat olive oil in a non-stick pan. Add chopped vegetables and sauté until tender.
3. Pour egg whites over the veggies. Cook until set, then fold the omelette in half.

**Nutritional Value:**
- High protein from egg whites.
- Veggies provide vitamins and minerals.
- Olive oil adds healthy fats.

**Cooking Time:** Around 10 minutes.

# 3. Cottage Cheese Pancakes

**Ingredients:**
- 1/2 cup low-fat cottage cheese
- 2 eggs
- 2 tablespoons almond flour
- 1/2 teaspoon vanilla extract
- Cooking spray

**Preparation:**

1. Blend cottage cheese, eggs, almond flour, and vanilla extract in a blender until smooth.

2. Heat a non-stick skillet and spray with cooking spray. Pour small circles of batter onto the skillet.

3. Cook until bubbles form, then flip and cook until golden brown.

**Nutritional Value:**
- High protein from cottage cheese and eggs.
- Almond flour adds a nutty flavor and healthy fats.

**Cooking Time:** Around 15 minutes.

# 4. Chia Seed Pudding

**Ingredients:**
- 2 tablespoons chia seeds
- 1/2 cup unsweetened almond milk
- 1/4 teaspoon vanilla extract
- 1/2 cup diced mixed fruit (e.g., kiwi, mango, or pineapple)

**Preparation:**
1. Mix chia seeds, almond milk, and vanilla extract in a bowl. Stir well.
2. Refrigerate for at least 2 hours or overnight, stirring occasionally.
3. Top with diced fruits before serving.

**- Nutritional Value:**
- Chia seeds are high in fiber and omega-3 fatty acids.
- Fruits offer vitamins and antioxidants.

**- Preparation Time:** Around 5 minutes (+ chilling time).

# 5. Greek Yogurt Parfait

**- Ingredients:**
  - 1/2 cup plain Greek yogurt
  - 2 tablespoons chopped nuts (e.g., walnuts or almonds)
  - 1/4 cup diced mixed berries
  - 1 teaspoon honey (optional)

**- Preparation:**
  1. Layer Greek yogurt, chopped nuts, and diced berries in a glass or bowl.
  2. Drizzle with honey if desired.

**- Nutritional Value:**
  - Greek yogurt provides protein and probiotics.
  - Nuts offer healthy fats and crunch.
  - Berries add antioxidants and vitamins.

**- Preparation Time:** Around 5 minutes.

# 6. Sweet Potato Breakfast Hash

**- Ingredients:**
  - 1 small sweet potato, diced
  - 1/4 cup diced bell peppers
  - 1/4 cup diced onions
  - 1 teaspoon olive oil
  - 2 eggs

- Salt and pepper to taste

**- Preparation:**

1. Heat olive oil in a skillet. Add diced sweet potatoes and cook until slightly tender.

2. Add bell peppers and onions, continue cooking until vegetables are cooked through.

3. Push veggies to the side, crack eggs into the skillet, and cook to desired doneness.

4. Season with salt and pepper before serving.

**- Nutritional Value:**
- Sweet potatoes offer vitamins and fiber.
- Eggs provide protein and essential nutrients.

**- Cooking Time:** Around 20 minutes.

# 7. Rice Cake with Avocado and Tomato

**- Ingredients:**
- 2 rice cakes
- 1/2 ripe avocado, mashed
- 1 small tomato, sliced
- Pinch of salt and black pepper

**- Preparation:**

1. Spread mashed avocado evenly over rice cakes.

2. Top with slices of tomato. Season with salt and black pepper.

**- Nutritional Value:**
  - Avocado provides healthy fats and potassium.
  - Tomatoes offer vitamins and antioxidants.

**- Preparation Time:** Around 5 minutes.

# 8. Oatmeal with Almond Butter and Banana

**- Ingredients:**
  - 1/2 cup rolled oats
  - 1 cup water or unsweetened almond milk
  - 1 tablespoon almond butter
  - 1 small banana, sliced

**- Preparation:**
1. Cook rolled oats with water or almond milk in a saucepan until creamy.
2. Transfer cooked oatmeal to a bowl. Top with almond butter and banana slices.

**- Nutritional Value:**
  - Oats are high in fiber and provide sustained energy.
  - Almond butter adds healthy fats and protein.
  - Bananas offer potassium and vitamins.

- **Cooking Time:** Around 10 minutes.

# 9. Egg Muffin Cups

- **Ingredients:**
  - 4 large eggs
  - 1/4 cup diced bell peppers
  - 1/4 cup diced spinach
  - Salt and pepper to taste
  - Cooking spray

- **Preparation:**
  1. Preheat oven to 350°F (175°C). Grease a muffin tin with cooking spray.
  2. In a bowl, whisk eggs and add diced vegetables, salt, and pepper.
  3. Pour the egg mixture evenly into the muffin cups.
  4. Bake for 15-18 minutes until the egg muffins are set.

- **Nutritional Value:**
  - High protein from eggs.
  - Veggies add vitamins and minerals.

- **Cooking Time:** Around 20 minutes.

# 10. Cottage Cheese and Fruit Salad

- **Ingredients:**
  - 1/2 cup low-fat cottage cheese
  - 1/2 cup diced mixed fruits (e.g., apples, grapes, oranges)
  - 1 tablespoon chopped nuts (optional)

- **Preparation:**
  1. Combine cottage cheese and diced fruits in a bowl.
  2. Sprinkle with chopped nuts if desired.

- **Nutritional Value:**
  - Cottage cheese offers protein and calcium.
  - Fruits provide vitamins and antioxidants.

- **Preparation Time:** Around 5 minutes.

# 11. Veggie Scramble

- **Ingredients:**
  - 2 eggs
  - 1/4 cup chopped mushrooms
  - 1/4 cup diced tomatoes
  - 1/4 cup chopped spinach
  - 1 teaspoon olive oil
  - Salt and pepper to taste

**- Preparation:**

1. Heat olive oil in a pan. Add mushrooms, tomatoes, and spinach. Sauté until vegetables are tender.

2. Whisk eggs and pour over the veggies. Cook until eggs are scrambled.

3. Season with salt and pepper before serving.

**- Nutritional Value:**
  - Eggs provide protein and essential nutrients.
  - Veggies offer vitamins and antioxidants.

**- Cooking Time:** Around 10 minutes.

# 12. Berry Smoothie Bowl

**- Ingredients:**
  - 1/2 cup frozen mixed berries
  - 1 ripe banana
  - 1/2 cup unsweetened almond milk
  - 2 tablespoons plain Greek yogurt
  - Toppings: sliced almonds, chia seeds (optional)

**- Preparation:**

1. Blend frozen berries, banana, almond milk, and Greek yogurt until smooth.

2. Pour into a bowl and add toppings like sliced almonds or chia seeds.

**- Nutritional Value:**

- Berries offer antioxidants and vitamins.
- Greek yogurt provides protein and probiotics.

- **Preparation Time:** Around 5 minutes.

# 13. Turkey and Veggie Wrap

- **Ingredients:**
  - 1 whole grain tortilla
  - 2 slices turkey breast
  - 1/4 cup shredded lettuce
  - 1/4 cup diced cucumber
  - 1 tablespoon hummus

- **Preparation:**
  1. Lay the tortilla flat. Spread hummus on it.
  2. Layer turkey slices, shredded lettuce, and diced cucumber.
  3. Roll the tortilla tightly into a wrap.

- **Nutritional Value:**
  - Turkey provides lean protein.
  - Veggies add vitamins and fiber.

- **Preparation Time:** Around 5 minutes.

# 14. Coconut Chia Seed Pudding

## - Ingredients:
- 2 tablespoons chia seeds
- 1/2 cup coconut milk
- 1/4 teaspoon vanilla extract
- 1 tablespoon shredded coconut

## - Preparation:
1. Mix chia seeds, coconut milk, and vanilla extract in a bowl. Stir well.
2. Refrigerate for at least 2 hours or overnight, stirring occasionally.
3. Top with shredded coconut before serving.

## - Nutritional Value:
- Chia seeds are high in fiber and omega-3 fatty acids.
- Coconut milk offers healthy fats and a tropical flavor.

## - Preparation Time: Around 5 minutes (+ chilling time).

# 15. Millet Porridge

## - Ingredients:
- 1/4 cup millet
- 1 cup water or unsweetened almond milk
- 1 tablespoon chopped nuts
- 1 tablespoon honey (optional)

## - Preparation:
1. Rinse millet. Cook millet with water or almond milk in a saucepan until soft.

2. Transfer to a bowl and top with chopped nuts. Add honey if desired.

## - Nutritional Value:
- Millet provides fiber and minerals.
- Nuts offer healthy fats and protein.

## - Cooking Time: Around 20-25 minutes.

# LUNCH RECIPES

## 1. Grilled Lemon Herb Chicken

### - Ingredients:
- 2 boneless, skinless chicken breasts
- 2 tablespoons olive oil
- 1 tablespoon lemon juice
- 1 teaspoon dried thyme
- 1 teaspoon dried rosemary
- Salt and pepper to taste

### - Preparation:
1. In a bowl, mix olive oil, lemon juice, thyme, rosemary, salt, and pepper to create a marinade.

2. Coat chicken breasts with the marinade. Let it sit for 15-20 minutes.

3. Heat a grill or grill pan over medium-high heat. Grill chicken for 6-7 minutes per side until fully cooked.

### - Nutritional Value:
- Chicken is a lean protein source.
- Herbs add flavor without excess sodium.
- Olive oil provides healthy fats.

### - Cooking Time: Around 15-20 minutes.

# 2. Salmon and Quinoa Salad

## - Ingredients:
- 2 salmon fillets
- 1 cup cooked quinoa
- 2 cups mixed greens
- 1/4 cup cherry tomatoes, halved
- 1/4 cup cucumber, sliced
- 2 tablespoons balsamic vinaigrette

## - Preparation:
1. Season salmon with salt and pepper. Grill or bake until cooked through.
2. In a bowl, toss mixed greens, cooked quinoa, cherry tomatoes, and cucumber with balsamic vinaigrette.
3. Top the salad with grilled salmon.

## - Nutritional Value:
- Salmon offers omega-3 fatty acids and protein.
- Quinoa provides fiber and essential nutrients.
- Vegetables add vitamins and antioxidants.

## - Cooking Time: Around 20 minutes.

# 3. Vegetable Stir-Fry with Tofu

## - Ingredients:
- 1 block firm tofu, pressed and cubed
- 2 cups mixed vegetables (bell peppers, broccoli, carrots)
- 2 tablespoons low-sodium soy sauce
- 1 tablespoon sesame oil
- 1 clove garlic, minced
- 1 teaspoon grated ginger
- Cooked brown rice (optional, for serving)

## - Preparation:
1. Heat sesame oil in a pan. Add minced garlic and grated ginger, sauté for a minute.
2. Add tofu cubes and stir-fry until lightly browned.
3. Add mixed vegetables and cook until tender-crisp.
4. Pour in low-sodium soy sauce, toss everything together.
5. Serve stir-fry alone or over cooked brown rice.

## - Nutritional Value:
- Tofu provides plant-based protein.
- Mixed vegetables offer vitamins and fiber.
- Brown rice adds complex carbs if included.

## - Cooking Time: Around 20 minutes.

# 4. Turkey and Veggie Lettuce Wraps

## - Ingredients:
- 1/2 lb. ground turkey
- 1 cup diced mixed vegetables (bell peppers, onions, carrots)
- 2 tablespoons low-sodium soy sauce
- 1 teaspoon olive oil
- Lettuce leaves for wrapping

## - Preparation:
1. Heat olive oil in a pan. Add ground turkey and cook until browned.
2. Add diced vegetables and sauté until softened.
3. Pour in low-sodium soy sauce, stir well.
4. Spoon the turkey and veggie mixture into lettuce leaves for wrapping.

## - Nutritional Value:
- Turkey offers lean protein.
- Mixed veggies provide vitamins and fiber.
- Lettuce wraps add crunch and reduce carb intake.

## - Cooking Time: Around 15 minutes.

# 5. Mediterranean Chickpea Salad

## - Ingredients:
- 1 can chickpeas, drained and rinsed
- 1 cucumber, diced
- 1 cup cherry tomatoes, halved
- 1/4 cup chopped red onion
- 2 tablespoons chopped fresh parsley
- 2 tablespoons olive oil
- 2 tablespoons lemon juice
- Salt and pepper to taste

## - Preparation:
1. In a bowl, combine chickpeas, cucumber, cherry tomatoes, red onion, and parsley.
2. Drizzle with olive oil and lemon juice. Season with salt and pepper, toss to combine.

## - Nutritional Value:
- Chickpeas offer plant-based protein and fiber.
- Vegetables provide vitamins and antioxidants.
- Olive oil adds healthy fats.

## - Preparation Time: Around 10 minutes.

# 6. Lemon Herb Baked Cod

## - Ingredients:
- 2 cod fillets
- 1 tablespoon olive oil
- 2 tablespoons lemon juice
- 1 teaspoon dried thyme
- 1 teaspoon dried parsley
- Salt and pepper to taste

## - Preparation:
1. Preheat oven to 375°F (190°C). Place cod fillets on a baking dish.
2. In a bowl, mix olive oil, lemon juice, thyme, parsley, salt, and pepper.
3. Drizzle the herb mixture over the cod fillets.
4. Bake for 15-20 minutes until the fish is cooked through.

## - Nutritional Value:
- Cod is a lean source of protein.
- Lemon and herbs add flavor without excess sodium.

## - Cooking Time: Around 15-20 minutes.

# 7. Vegetable Lentil Soup

## - Ingredients:
- 1 cup dried green or brown lentils, rinsed
- 4 cups low-sodium vegetable broth
- 1 cup diced carrots
- 1 cup diced celery
- 1 cup diced onions
- 2 cloves garlic, minced
- 1 teaspoon dried thyme
- Salt and pepper to taste

## - Preparation:
1. In a large pot, combine lentils, vegetable broth, carrots, celery, onions, garlic, thyme, salt, and pepper.
2. Bring to a boil, then reduce heat and simmer for 25-30 minutes until lentils and vegetables are tender.

## - Nutritional Value:
- Lentils offer plant-based protein and fiber.
- Vegetables provide vitamins and minerals.

## - Cooking Time: Around 30 minutes.

# 8. Tuna Salad Lettuce Wraps

## - Ingredients:
- 2 cans (5 oz. each) tuna, drained
- 1/4 cup diced red bell pepper
- 1/4 cup diced cucumber
- 2 tablespoons chopped fresh parsley
- 2 tablespoons olive oil
- 1 tablespoon lemon juice
- Lettuce leaves for wrapping

## - Preparation:
1. In a bowl, mix tuna, diced bell pepper, cucumber, parsley, olive oil, and lemon juice.
2. Spoon the tuna salad into lettuce leaves for wrapping.

## - Nutritional Value:
- Tuna provides protein and omega-3 fatty acids.
- Bell pepper and cucumber offer vitamins and antioxidants.

## - Preparation Time: Around 10 minutes.

# 9. Chicken and Vegetable Skewers

## - Ingredients:
- 2 boneless, skinless chicken breasts, cut into cubes
- 1 zucchini, sliced
- 1 bell pepper, diced
- 1 red onion, cut into chunks
- 2 tablespoons olive oil
- 1 teaspoon paprika
- Salt and pepper to taste

## - Preparation:
1. Preheat grill or grill pan over medium-high heat.
2. Thread chicken cubes, zucchini slices, bell pepper, and onion chunks onto skewers.
3. In a bowl, mix olive oil, paprika, salt, and pepper. Brush the skewers with this mixture.
4. Grill skewers for 10-12 minutes, turning occasionally, until chicken is cooked through.

## - Nutritional Value:
- Chicken provides lean protein.
- Vegetables offer vitamins and fiber.

## - Cooking Time: Around 15 minutes.

# 10. Eggplant and Tomato Stew

## - Ingredients:
- 1 large eggplant, diced
- 2 cups diced tomatoes (canned or fresh)
- 1 onion, diced
- 2 cloves garlic, minced
- 1 teaspoon dried oregano
- 1 teaspoon olive oil
- Salt and pepper to taste

## - Preparation:
1. Heat olive oil in a pot. Add onion and garlic, sauté until softened.

2. Add diced eggplant, tomatoes, dried oregano, salt, and pepper. Stir well.

3. Simmer for 20-25 minutes until the eggplant is tender and flavors meld.

## - Nutritional Value:
- Eggplant offers fiber and antioxidants.
- Tomatoes provide vitamins and lycopene.

## - Cooking Time: Around 25 minutes.

# 11. Mushroom and Spinach Quinoa

## - Ingredients:
- 1 cup quinoa, rinsed
- 2 cups low-sodium vegetable broth
- 1 tablespoon olive oil
- 1 cup sliced mushrooms
- 2 cups fresh spinach
- Salt and pepper to taste

## - Preparation:
1. In a pot, combine quinoa and vegetable broth. Bring to a boil, then reduce heat and simmer for 15-20 minutes until quinoa is cooked and liquid is absorbed.

2. In a separate pan, heat olive oil. Sauté mushrooms until they release moisture, then add spinach and cook until wilted.

3. Combine cooked quinoa with the mushroom and spinach mixture. Season with salt and pepper.

## - Nutritional Value:
- Quinoa offers protein and fiber.
- Spinach provides vitamins and minerals.
- Mushrooms add flavor and nutrients.

## - Cooking Time: Around 25 minutes.

# 12. Turkey and Vegetable Stir-Fry

- **Ingredients:**
  - 1/2 lb. ground turkey
  - 2 cups mixed vegetables (broccoli, bell peppers, snap peas)
  - 2 tablespoons low-sodium soy sauce
  - 1 tablespoon olive oil
  - 2 cloves garlic, minced
  - Cooked brown rice (optional, for serving)

- **Preparation:**
  1. Heat olive oil in a skillet. Add minced garlic and cook for a minute.
  2. Add ground turkey and cook until browned.
  3. Add mixed vegetables and stir-fry until tender.
  4. Pour in low-sodium soy sauce, stir well.
  5. Serve stir-fry alone or over cooked brown rice.

- **Nutritional Value:**
  - Turkey offers lean protein.
  - Mixed vegetables provide vitamins and fiber.
  - Brown rice adds optional complex carbs.

- **Cooking Time:** Around 20 minutes.

# 13. Vegetarian Bean Burrito Bowl

## - Ingredients:
- 1 cup cooked brown rice
- 1 cup black beans, drained and rinsed
- 1 cup corn kernels (fresh or frozen)
- 1/2 cup diced tomatoes
- 1/4 cup chopped cilantro
- 1/4 cup diced avocado
- Squeeze of lime juice
- Optional: salsa or hot sauce

## - Preparation:
1. Divide cooked brown rice among serving bowls.
2. Top with black beans, corn kernels, diced tomatoes, chopped cilantro, and diced avocado.
3. Squeeze lime juice over the bowl and add salsa or hot sauce if desired.

## - Nutritional Value:
- Brown rice offers fiber and nutrients.
- Black beans provide plant-based protein and fiber.
- Avocado adds healthy fats and creaminess.

## - Preparation Time: Around 10 minutes.

# 14. Roasted Vegetable Quiche

**- Ingredients:**
  - 1 prepared pie crust (store-bought or homemade)
  - 1 cup mixed roasted vegetables (zucchini, bell peppers, onions)
  - 4 eggs
  - 1 cup low-fat milk
  - 1/2 cup shredded cheese (optional)
  - Salt and pepper to taste

**- Preparation:**
  1. Preheat oven to 375°F (190°C). Place roasted vegetables in the pie crust.
  2. In a bowl, whisk together eggs, milk, shredded cheese (if using), salt, and pepper.
  3. Pour egg mixture over the roasted vegetables in the pie crust.
  4. Bake for 35-40 minutes until the quiche is set and golden brown.

**- Nutritional Value:**
  - Eggs provide protein and essential nutrients.
  - Roasted vegetables offer vitamins and fiber.

**- Cooking Time:** Around 45 minutes.

# 15. Chicken and Avocado Salad

**- Ingredients:**
- 2 cups cooked chicken breast, shredded or diced
- 1 avocado, diced
- 1 cup mixed greens
- 1/4 cup diced red onion
- 2 tablespoons chopped fresh parsley
- 2 tablespoons olive oil
- 1 tablespoon lemon juice
- Salt and pepper to taste

**- Preparation:**
1. In a bowl, combine cooked chicken, diced avocado, mixed greens, diced red onion, and chopped parsley.
2. In a separate small bowl, whisk together olive oil, lemon juice, salt, and pepper to make the dressing.
3. Drizzle the dressing over the salad and toss gently to combine.

**- Nutritional Value:**
- Chicken provides protein.
- Avocado adds healthy fats and creaminess.
- Mixed greens offer vitamins and minerals.

**- Preparation Time:** Around 10 minutes.

# DINNER RECIPES

## 1. Baked Lemon Herb Salmon

**- Ingredients:**
  - 2 salmon fillets
  - 2 tablespoons olive oil
  - 2 tablespoons lemon juice
  - 1 teaspoon dried dill
  - 1 teaspoon dried parsley
  - Salt and pepper to taste

**- Preparation:**
  1. Preheat oven to 375°F (190°C). Place salmon fillets on a baking dish.
  2. In a bowl, mix olive oil, lemon juice, dried dill, dried parsley, salt, and pepper.
  3. Drizzle the herb mixture over the salmon fillets.
  4. Bake for 12-15 minutes until the fish is cooked through.

**- Nutritional Value:**
  - Salmon offers omega-3 fatty acids and protein.
  - Lemon and herbs add flavor without excess sodium.

**- Cooking Time:** Around 15 minutes.

# 2. Turkey Chili

## - Ingredients:
- 1 lb. ground turkey
- 1 can (15 oz.) low-sodium kidney beans, drained and rinsed
- 1 can (15 oz.) diced tomatoes
- 1 cup low-sodium chicken or vegetable broth
- 1 cup diced bell peppers
- 1 cup diced onions
- 2 cloves garlic, minced
- 2 tablespoons chili powder
- 1 teaspoon cumin
- Salt and pepper to taste

## - Preparation:
1. In a pot, brown ground turkey over medium heat. Drain excess fat.
2. Add diced onions, bell peppers, and garlic. Cook until vegetables soften.
3. Stir in diced tomatoes, kidney beans, chicken or vegetable broth, chili powder, cumin, salt, and pepper.
4. Simmer for 20-25 minutes, stirring occasionally.

## - Nutritional Value:
- Turkey offers lean protein.
- Kidney beans provide plant-based protein and fiber.
- Vegetables add vitamins and minerals.

- **Cooking Time:** Around 30 minutes.

# 3. Grilled Chicken and Vegetable Kabobs

- **Ingredients:**
  - 2 boneless, skinless chicken breasts, cut into cubes
  - 1 zucchini, sliced
  - 1 bell pepper, diced
  - 1 red onion, cut into chunks
  - 2 tablespoons olive oil
  - 1 teaspoon paprika
  - Salt and pepper to taste

- **Preparation:**
  1. Preheat grill or grill pan over medium-high heat.
  2. Thread chicken cubes, zucchini slices, bell pepper, and onion chunks onto skewers.
  3. In a bowl, mix olive oil, paprika, salt, and pepper. Brush the skewers with this mixture.
  4. Grill skewers for 10-12 minutes, turning occasionally, until chicken is cooked through.

- **Nutritional Value:**
  - Chicken provides protein.
  - Vegetables offer vitamins and fiber.
  - Olive oil adds healthy fats.

- **Cooking Time:** Around 15 minutes.

# 4. Vegetarian Lentil Curry

## - Ingredients:
- 1 cup dried lentils, rinsed
- 2 cups low-sodium vegetable broth
- 1 can (15 oz.) diced tomatoes
- 1 cup chopped spinach
- 1 cup diced carrots
- 1 onion, diced
- 2 cloves garlic, minced
- 1 tablespoon olive oil
- 2 tablespoons curry powder
- Salt and pepper to taste

## - Preparation:
1. In a pot, heat olive oil. Sauté onions and garlic until softened.
2. Add diced carrots, lentils, diced tomatoes, vegetable broth, curry powder, salt, and pepper.
3. Bring to a boil, then reduce heat and simmer for 25-30 minutes until lentils are tender.
4. Stir in chopped spinach and cook for an additional 5 minutes.

## - Nutritional Value:
- Lentils offer plant-based protein and fiber.
- Vegetables provide vitamins and minerals.

- Spinach adds nutrients and flavor.

- **Cooking Time:** Around 35 minutes.

# 5. Baked Herb Chicken with Roasted Vegetables

- **Ingredients:**
  - 2 boneless, skinless chicken breasts
  - 2 tablespoons olive oil
  - 1 teaspoon dried thyme
  - 1 teaspoon dried rosemary
  - 2 cups mixed vegetables (zucchini, bell peppers, onions)
  - Salt and pepper to taste

- **Preparation:**
  1. Preheat oven to 400°F (200°C). Place chicken breasts on a baking dish.
  2. In a bowl, mix olive oil, dried thyme, dried rosemary, salt, and pepper.
  3. Rub the herb mixture over the chicken breasts.
  4. Place mixed vegetables around the chicken on the baking dish.
  5. Bake for 20-25 minutes until the chicken is cooked through and vegetables are tender.

- **Nutritional Value:**
  - Chicken offers protein.

- Mixed vegetables provide vitamins and fiber.
- Olive oil adds healthy fats.

- **Cooking Time:** Around 25 minutes.

# 6. Quinoa and Vegetable Stir-Fry

## - Ingredients:
- 1 cup quinoa, rinsed
- 2 cups low-sodium vegetable broth
- 1 tablespoon olive oil
- 2 cups mixed vegetables (broccoli, bell peppers, carrots)
- 2 cloves garlic, minced
- 2 tablespoons low-sodium soy sauce
- Salt and pepper to taste

## - Preparation:
1. In a pot, cook quinoa in vegetable broth according to package instructions.
2. Heat olive oil in a pan. Sauté minced garlic until fragrant.
3. Add mixed vegetables and stir-fry until tender.
4. Add cooked quinoa to the pan and stir in low-sodium soy sauce. Mix well.
5. Season with salt and pepper to taste.

## - Nutritional Value:
- Quinoa provides protein and fiber.
- Mixed vegetables offer vitamins and minerals.
- Olive oil adds healthy fats.

- **Cooking Time:** Around 25 minutes.

# 7. Lemon Garlic Shrimp Pasta

- **Ingredients:**
    - 8 oz whole grain pasta
    - 1 lb shrimp, peeled and deveined
    - 2 tablespoons olive oil
    - 3 cloves garlic, minced
    - Zest and juice of 1 lemon
    - 1/4 cup chopped fresh parsley
    - Salt and pepper to taste

- **Preparation:**
    1. Cook pasta according to package instructions.
    2. In a skillet, heat olive oil. Add minced garlic and cook until fragrant.
    3. Add shrimp and cook until pink and cooked through.
    4. Toss cooked pasta with lemon zest, lemon juice, chopped parsley, cooked shrimp, and garlic oil.
    5. Season with salt and pepper.

- **Nutritional Value:**
    - Shrimp provides protein.
    - Whole grain pasta offers fiber and nutrients.
    - Olive oil and garlic add flavor without excess sodium.

- **Cooking Time:** Around 20 minutes.

# 8. Tofu and Broccoli Stir-Fry

## - Ingredients:
- 1 block firm tofu, pressed and cubed
- 2 cups broccoli florets
- 2 tablespoons low-sodium soy sauce
- 1 tablespoon sesame oil
- 1 tablespoon honey
- 2 cloves garlic, minced
- Cooked brown rice (optional, for serving)

## - Preparation:
1. In a bowl, mix low-sodium soy sauce, sesame oil, and honey.
2. Heat a pan or wok. Add minced garlic and sauté until fragrant.
3. Add cubed tofu and cook until lightly browned.
4. Add broccoli florets and stir-fry until tender-crisp.
5. Pour in the soy sauce mixture and toss everything together.
6. Serve over cooked brown rice if desired.

## - Nutritional Value:
- Tofu provides plant-based protein.
- Broccoli offers vitamins and fiber.
- Brown rice adds optional complex carbs.

## - Cooking Time: Around 20 minutes.

# 9. Baked Chicken Fajitas

## - Ingredients:
- 1 lb boneless, skinless chicken breasts, sliced
- 2 bell peppers, sliced
- 1 onion, sliced
- 2 tablespoons olive oil
- 1 tablespoon chili powder
- 1 teaspoon cumin
- Salt and pepper to taste
- Whole wheat tortillas (optional, for serving)

## - Preparation:
1. Preheat oven to 400°F (200°C). Line a baking sheet with parchment paper.
2. Place sliced chicken, bell peppers, and onion on the baking sheet.
3. Drizzle with olive oil and sprinkle chili powder, cumin, salt, and pepper. Toss to coat evenly.
4. Bake for 20-25 minutes until chicken is cooked through and vegetables are tender.
5. Serve with whole wheat tortillas if desired.

## - Nutritional Value:
- Chicken offers protein.
- Bell peppers and onions provide vitamins and antioxidants.
- Olive oil adds healthy fats.

- **Cooking Time:** Around 25 minutes.

# 10. Mediterranean Veggie and Tuna Salad

- **Ingredients:**
  - 2 cans (5 oz each) tuna, drained
  - 1 cup diced cucumber
  - 1 cup cherry tomatoes, halved
  - 1/4 cup diced red onion
  - 1/4 cup chopped Kalamata olives
  - 2 tablespoons chopped fresh parsley
  - 2 tablespoons olive oil
  - 2 tablespoons lemon juice
  - Salt and pepper to taste

- **Preparation:**
  1. In a large bowl, combine tuna, diced cucumber, cherry tomatoes, red onion, Kalamata olives, and chopped parsley.
  2. In a small bowl, whisk together olive oil, lemon juice, salt, and pepper to make the dressing.
  3. Drizzle the dressing over the salad and toss gently to combine.

- **Nutritional Value:**
  - Tuna offers protein and omega-3 fatty acids.
  - Vegetables provide vitamins and antioxidants.

- Olive oil adds healthy fats and flavor.

- **Preparation Time:** Around 10 minutes.

# 11. Lemon Herb Baked Chicken

- **Ingredients:**
  - 4 boneless, skinless chicken breasts
  - 2 tablespoons olive oil
  - Zest and juice of 1 lemon
  - 2 cloves garlic, minced
  - 1 teaspoon dried thyme
  - 1 teaspoon dried rosemary
  - Salt and pepper to taste

- **Preparation:**
  1. Preheat oven to 375°F (190°C). Place chicken breasts in a baking dish.
  2. In a bowl, combine olive oil, lemon zest, lemon juice, minced garlic, dried thyme, dried rosemary, salt, and pepper.
  3. Pour the mixture over the chicken breasts, ensuring they're evenly coated.
  4. Bake for 20-25 minutes or until the chicken is cooked through.

- **Nutritional Value:**
  - Chicken provides protein.
  - Lemon and herbs add flavor without excess sodium.

- **Cooking Time:** Around 25 minutes.

# 12. Turkey Meatballs with Marinara Sauce

## - Ingredients:
- 1 lb. ground turkey
- 1/4 cup breadcrumbs (ensure low phosphorus)
- 1/4 cup grated Parmesan cheese (optional)
- 1 egg
- 2 cloves garlic, minced
- 2 cups low-sodium marinara sauce
- 1 teaspoon dried basil
- 1 teaspoon dried oregano
- Salt and pepper to taste

## - Preparation:
1. Preheat oven to 375°F (190°C). Line a baking sheet with parchment paper.
2. In a bowl, combine ground turkey, breadcrumbs, Parmesan cheese (if using), egg, minced garlic, salt, and pepper. Form into meatballs.
3. Place meatballs on the prepared baking sheet and bake for 20-25 minutes.
4. In a saucepan, heat marinara sauce with dried basil and dried oregano. Add the baked meatballs to the sauce and simmer for a few minutes before serving.

- **Nutritional Value:**
  - Turkey provides lean protein.
  - Marinara sauce offers vitamins from tomatoes.
  - Herbs add flavor without excess sodium.

- **Cooking Time:** Around 25 minutes.

# 13. Eggplant Parmesan

- **Ingredients:**
  - 2 medium eggplants, sliced
  - 1 cup whole grain breadcrumbs
  - 1/2 cup grated Parmesan cheese (optional)
  - 2 eggs, beaten
  - 2 cups low-sodium marinara sauce
  - 1 cup shredded mozzarella cheese
  - 2 tablespoons olive oil
  - Salt and pepper to taste

- **Preparation:**
  1. Preheat oven to 375°F (190°C). Line a baking sheet with parchment paper.
  2. Dip eggplant slices in beaten eggs, then coat with breadcrumbs and Parmesan cheese (if using).
  3. Place coated eggplant slices on the baking sheet. Drizzle with olive oil and bake for 20-25 minutes until golden.
  4. In a baking dish, layer baked eggplant slices, marinara sauce, and shredded mozzarella cheese. Repeat layers.

5. Bake for an additional 20 minutes until bubbly and cheese is melted.

**- Nutritional Value:**
   - Eggplant offers fiber and antioxidants.
   - Whole grain breadcrumbs provide fiber.
   - Cheeses offer protein and calcium (if included).

**- Cooking Time:** Around 45-50 minutes.

# 14. Lemon Garlic Shrimp Stir-Fry

**- Ingredients:**
   - 1 lb. shrimp, peeled and deveined
   - 2 cups mixed vegetables (bell peppers, broccoli, snap peas)
   - 2 tablespoons low-sodium soy sauce
   - 2 tablespoons olive oil
   - 3 cloves garlic, minced
   - Zest and juice of 1 lemon
   - Cooked brown rice (optional, for serving)

**- Preparation:**
   1. In a bowl, combine shrimp with low-sodium soy sauce, minced garlic, lemon zest, and lemon juice. Marinate for 10 minutes.
   2. Heat olive oil in a skillet or wok. Stir-fry marinated shrimp for 2-3 minutes until pink, then remove from the pan.

3. Add mixed vegetables to the same pan and stir-fry until tender-crisp.

4. Return cooked shrimp to the pan, toss everything together, and cook for an additional minute.

5. Serve over cooked brown rice if desired.

**- Nutritional Value:**
- Shrimp provides protein.
- Mixed vegetables offer vitamins and fiber.
- Brown rice adds optional complex carbs.

**- Cooking Time:** Around 20 minutes.

# 15. Herb-Roasted Vegetables

**- Ingredients**:
- 4 cups assorted vegetables (bell peppers, zucchini, cherry tomatoes, onions)
- 2 tablespoons olive oil
- 1 teaspoon dried thyme
- 1 teaspoon dried rosemary
- Salt and pepper to taste

**- Preparation:**
1. Preheat oven to 400°F (200°C). Line a baking sheet with parchment paper.

2. Cut vegetables into bite-sized pieces and place them on the baking sheet.

3. Drizzle olive oil over the vegetables and sprinkle with dried thyme, dried rosemary, salt, and pepper. Toss to coat evenly.

4. Roast in the oven for 20-25 minutes or until vegetables are tender and slightly browned.

### - Nutritional Value:
- Assorted vegetables offer vitamins, minerals, and fiber.
- Olive oil provides healthy fats.

### - Cooking Time: Around 25 minutes.

# SNACKS RECIPES

## 1. Baked Zucchini Chips

**- Ingredients:**
- 2 medium zucchinis, thinly sliced
- 2 tablespoons olive oil
- Salt and pepper to taste

**- Preparation:**
1. Preheat oven to 225°F (110°C). Line a baking sheet with parchment paper.
2. Place the zucchini slices on the baking sheet.
3. Drizzle olive oil over the slices and sprinkle with salt and pepper.
4. Bake for 2-3 hours until the zucchini slices are crispy, flipping them halfway through.

**- Nutritional Value:**
- Zucchini offers vitamins and minerals.
- Olive oil provides healthy fats.

**- Cooking Time:** Around 2-3 hours.

# 2. Hummus with Veggie Sticks

## - Ingredients:
- 1 can (15 oz.) low-sodium chickpeas, drained and rinsed
- 2 tablespoons olive oil
- 2 tablespoons tahini
- Juice of 1 lemon
- 2 cloves garlic, minced
- Salt and pepper to taste
- Assorted vegetable sticks (carrots, cucumber, bell peppers) for dipping

## - Preparation:
1. In a food processor, blend chickpeas, olive oil, tahini, lemon juice, minced garlic, salt, and pepper until smooth.
2. Serve the hummus with assorted vegetable sticks for dipping.

## - Nutritional Value:
- Chickpeas offer protein and fiber.
- Vegetables provide vitamins and minerals.

## - Preparation Time: Around 10 minutes.

# 3. Cottage Cheese and Berry Parfait

## - Ingredients:
- 1 cup low-fat cottage cheese
- 1/2 cup mixed berries (strawberries, blueberries, raspberries)
- 2 tablespoons chopped nuts (almonds, walnuts)
- 1 teaspoon honey (optional)

## - Preparation:
1. In a serving glass or bowl, layer low-fat cottage cheese, mixed berries, and chopped nuts.
2. Drizzle with honey if desired.

## - Nutritional Value:
- Cottage cheese offers protein and calcium.
- Berries provide antioxidants and fiber.
- Nuts add healthy fats and nutrients.

## - Preparation Time: Around 5 minutes.

# 4. Baked Sweet Potato Fries

## - Ingredients:
- 2 medium sweet potatoes, peeled and cut into strips
- 2 tablespoons olive oil
- 1 teaspoon paprika
- 1 teaspoon garlic powder
- Salt and pepper to taste

## - Preparation:
1. Preheat oven to 425°F (220°C). Line a baking sheet with parchment paper.

2. In a bowl, toss sweet potato strips with olive oil, paprika, garlic powder, salt, and pepper.

3. Spread the seasoned sweet potatoes in a single layer on the baking sheet.

4. Bake for 20-25 minutes until fries are crispy and golden, flipping them halfway through.

## - Nutritional Value:
- Sweet potatoes offer vitamins and fiber.
- Olive oil provides healthy fats.

## - Cooking Time: Around 20-25 minutes.

## - Nutritional Value:
- Greek yogurt offers protein and calcium.
- Mixed fruits provide vitamins and antioxidants.

# 5. Egg Salad Lettuce Wraps

## - Ingredients:
- 4 hard-boiled eggs, peeled and chopped
- 2 tablespoons low-fat mayonnaise
- 1 tablespoon Dijon mustard
- 1 stalk celery, finely chopped
- 2 tablespoons chopped chives or green onions
- Salt and pepper to taste
- Large lettuce leaves for wrapping

## - Preparation:
1. In a bowl, combine chopped hard-boiled eggs, low-fat mayonnaise, Dijon mustard, chopped celery, chopped chives or green onions, salt, and pepper.
2. Spoon the egg salad onto large lettuce leaves and wrap them like a burrito.

## - Nutritional Value:
- Eggs offer protein and nutrients.
- Lettuce provides a low-calorie base.
- Celery adds crunch and fiber.

## - Preparation Time: Around 15 minutes.

# 6. Cucumber Tuna Boats

## - Ingredients:
- 2 large cucumbers
- 2 cans (5 oz. each) tuna, drained
- 2 tablespoons low-fat mayonnaise or Greek yogurt
- 1 tablespoon lemon juice
- 1/4 cup diced red onion
- 1/4 cup diced bell peppers
- Salt and pepper to taste

## - Preparation:
1. Cut the cucumbers in half lengthwise and scoop out the seeds to create a "boat" shape.
2. In a bowl, mix drained tuna, low-fat mayonnaise or Greek yogurt, lemon juice, diced red onion, diced bell peppers, salt, and pepper.
3. Fill each cucumber boat with the tuna mixture.

## - Nutritional Value:
- Tuna offers protein and omega-3 fatty acids.
- Cucumbers provide hydration and vitamins.
- Bell peppers and onions add flavor and nutrients.

## - Preparation Time: Around 15 minutes.

# DESSERTS AND TREATS RECIPES

## 1. Mixed Berry Frozen Yogurt Popsicles

**- Ingredients:**
- 1 cup mixed berries (strawberries, blueberries, raspberries)
- 2 cups low-fat Greek yogurt
- 2 tablespoons honey (optional)

**- Preparation:**
1. Blend mixed berries in a food processor or blender until smooth.
2. In a bowl, mix blended berries with low-fat Greek yogurt and honey (if using).
3. Pour the mixture into popsicle molds.
4. Freeze for at least 4-6 hours until solid.

**- Nutritional Value:**
- Greek yogurt offers protein and calcium.
- Berries provide antioxidants and vitamins.

**- Preparation Time:** Around 10 minutes + freezing time.

# 2. Baked Apple Slices

## - Ingredients:
- 2 apples, cored and sliced
- 1 tablespoon unsalted butter or margarine
- 1 teaspoon cinnamon
- 1 tablespoon brown sugar (optional)

## - Preparation:
1. Preheat oven to 350°F (175°C). Line a baking sheet with parchment paper.
2. Arrange apple slices on the baking sheet.
3. Dot apple slices with unsalted butter or margarine.
4. Sprinkle cinnamon and brown sugar (if using) over the apples.
5. Bake for 20-25 minutes until apples are tender.

## - Nutritional Value:
- Apples offer fiber and nutrients.
- Cinnamon adds flavor without added sugar.

## - Cooking Time: Around 20-25 minutes.

# 3. Banana Oat Cookies

## - Ingredients:
- 2 ripe bananas, mashed
- 1 cup old-fashioned oats
- 1/4 cup chopped nuts (walnuts, almonds)
- 1/4 cup raisins or dried cranberries
- 1 teaspoon cinnamon
- 1/2 teaspoon vanilla extract

## - Preparation:
1. Preheat oven to 350°F (175°C). Line a baking sheet with parchment paper.

2. In a bowl, combine mashed bananas, oats, chopped nuts, raisins or dried cranberries, cinnamon, and vanilla extract.

3. Drop spoonful's of the mixture onto the baking sheet.

4. Flatten slightly with a fork and bake for 15-20 minutes until golden.

## - Nutritional Value:
- Bananas provide potassium and fiber.
- Oats offer fiber and nutrients.
- Nuts add healthy fats and protein.

## - Cooking Time: Around 15-20 minutes.

# 4. Coconut Milk Rice Pudding

## - Ingredients:
- 1 cup cooked white rice
- 2 cups unsweetened coconut milk
- 1/4 cup honey or maple syrup (optional)
- 1 teaspoon vanilla extract
- Ground cinnamon for garnish (optional)

## - Preparation:
1. In a saucepan, combine cooked rice, unsweetened coconut milk, honey or maple syrup (if using), and vanilla extract.

2. Cook over medium heat, stirring occasionally, until thickened (approximately 20-25 minutes).

3. Remove from heat and let it cool. Refrigerate before serving.

4. Sprinkle with ground cinnamon if desired.

## - Nutritional Value:
- Coconut milk provides a creamy texture.
- Rice offers carbohydrates and calories.

## - Cooking Time: Around 25 minutes.

# 5. Frozen Banana Bites

## - Ingredients:
- 2 ripe bananas
- 1/4 cup dark chocolate chips (unsweetened if possible)
- 1 tablespoon coconut oil
- Chopped nuts or shredded coconut for topping (optional)

## - Preparation:
1. Line a baking sheet with parchment paper.
2. Slice bananas into rounds and place them on the prepared baking sheet.
3. Melt dark chocolate chips and coconut oil together in the microwave or using a double boiler.
4. Dip each banana slice halfway into the melted chocolate mixture.
5. Sprinkle chopped nuts or shredded coconut on top if desired.
6. Place in the freezer for 1-2 hours until the chocolate hardens.

## - Nutritional Value:
- Bananas offer potassium and fiber.
- Dark chocolate provides antioxidants.

## - Preparation Time: Around 10 minutes + freezing time.

# 6. Vanilla Yogurt with Fresh Berries

## - Ingredients:
- 1 cup low-fat vanilla yogurt
- 1/2 cup mixed fresh berries (strawberries, blueberries, raspberries)

## - Preparation:
1. Spoon low-fat vanilla yogurt into a serving bowl.
2. Top with mixed fresh berries.

## - Nutritional Value:
- Low-fat vanilla yogurt offers protein and calcium.
- Berries provide antioxidants and vitamins.

## - Preparation Time: Around 2-3 minutes.

# BEVERAGES AND DRINKS RECIPES

## 1. Herbal Infused Water

**- Ingredients:**
- 1 liter water
- Fresh herbs (such as mint, basil, or rosemary)
- Sliced fruits (such as lemon, lime, or cucumber)
- Ice cubes (optional)

**- Preparation:**
1. Fill a pitcher with water.
2. Add fresh herbs and sliced fruits to the water.
3. Refrigerate for at least 2 hours or overnight to allow the flavors to infuse.
4. Serve over ice cubes if desired.

**- Nutritional Value:**
- Hydrating and refreshing.
- Herbs and fruits offer vitamins and antioxidants.

**- Preparation Time:** Around 5 minutes (+ infusing time).

# 2. Green Tea with Lemon

**- Ingredients:**
  - 1 green tea bag
  - 1 cup hot water
  - Squeeze of fresh lemon juice
  - Honey or stevia (optional, for sweetness)

**- Preparation:**
  1. Steep a green tea bag in hot water for 3-5 minutes.
  2. Remove the tea bag and add a squeeze of fresh lemon juice.
  3. Sweeten with honey or stevia if desired.

**- Nutritional Value:**
  - Green tea offers antioxidants.
  - Lemon provides vitamin C.

**- Preparation Time:** Around 5 minutes.

# 3. Watermelon Mint Smoothie

**- Ingredients:**
  - 2 cups diced watermelon (seedless)
  - 1/2 cup plain low-fat yogurt
  - 4-5 fresh mint leaves
  - 1 teaspoon honey (optional)
  - Ice cubes (optional)

**- Preparation:**

1. Place diced watermelon, low-fat yogurt, fresh mint leaves, and honey (if using) in a blender.

2. Blend until smooth.

3. Add ice cubes if a colder consistency is desired and blend again.

**- Nutritional Value:**
- Watermelon provides hydration and vitamins.
- Yogurt offers protein and calcium.
- Mint adds a refreshing flavor.

**- Preparation Time:** Around 5 minutes.

# 4. Golden Milk (Turmeric Latte)

**- Ingredients:**
- 1 cup unsweetened almond milk (or any preferred milk)
- 1/2 teaspoon ground turmeric
- 1/4 teaspoon ground cinnamon
- 1/4 teaspoon ground ginger
- Pinch of black pepper (to enhance turmeric absorption)
- 1 teaspoon honey or maple syrup (optional)

**- Preparation:**

1. In a small saucepan, heat almond milk over medium-low heat.

2. Whisk in ground turmeric, ground cinnamon, ground ginger, black pepper, and honey or maple syrup (if using).

3. Heat for a few minutes, stirring constantly until warm but not boiling.

4. Pour into a cup and serve.

**- Nutritional Value:**
   - Turmeric provides anti-inflammatory properties.
   - Almond milk offers a dairy-free base.

**- Preparation Time:** Around 5 minutes.

# 5. Berry Spinach Smoothie

**- Ingredients:**
   - 1/2 cup frozen mixed berries
   - 1 handful fresh spinach leaves
   - 1/2 cup low-fat Greek yogurt
   - 1/2 cup unsweetened almond milk (or any preferred milk)
   - 1 tablespoon chia seeds (optional)

**- Preparation:**
1. Place frozen mixed berries, fresh spinach leaves, low-fat Greek yogurt, unsweetened almond milk, and chia seeds (if using) in a blender.

2. Blend until smooth.

**- Nutritional Value:**
   - Berries provide antioxidants and vitamins.

- Spinach offers nutrients and fiber.
- Greek yogurt adds protein and calcium.

- **Preparation Time:** Around 5 minutes.

# 6. Pineapple Ginger Cooler

- **Ingredients:**
  - 1 cup fresh pineapple chunks
  - 1 teaspoon grated fresh ginger
  - 1 cup coconut water
  - 1 teaspoon honey or agave syrup (optional)
  - Ice cubes (optional)

- **Preparation:**
1. In a blender, combine fresh pineapple chunks, grated fresh ginger, coconut water, and honey or agave syrup (if using).
2. Blend until smooth.
3. Add ice cubes if desired and blend again.

- **Nutritional Value:**
  - Pineapple provides vitamins and enzymes.
  - Ginger offers digestive benefits.
  - Coconut water offers hydration and electrolytes.

- **Preparation Time:** Around 5 minutes.

# 7. Cranberry Iced Tea

## - Ingredients:

- 2 cups unsweetened cranberry juice
- 2 cups water
- 2 tea bags (black tea or herbal tea of choice)
- Ice cubes
- Fresh lemon slices for garnish (optional)

## - Preparation:

1. Boil 2 cups of water and steep the tea bags for 3-5 minutes.

2. In a pitcher, mix unsweetened cranberry juice and brewed tea.

3. Allow the mixture to cool, then refrigerate.

4. Serve the cranberry iced tea over ice cubes in glasses.

Garnish with fresh lemon slices if desired.

## Nutritional Value:

Cranberry juice offers antioxidants and vitamins.
Tea provides flavonoids and potential health benefits.
Lemon adds vitamin C and flavor.

**Preparation Time:** Around 15 minutes.

# CONCLUSION

In conclusion, this CKD Stage 4 cookbook for seniors serves as a valuable resource, offering a comprehensive array of kidney-friendly recipes and essential dietary guidelines tailored to manage chronic kidney disease effectively. With a focus on nutrient balance and restriction of phosphorus, potassium, sodium, and protein, these recipes aim to slow disease progression, alleviate symptoms, and promote optimal health.

The diverse range of recipes encompasses protein sources like poultry and fish, alongside fruits and vegetables low in potassium, phosphorus, and sodium. Incorporating healthy fats, grains, dairy substitutes, and carefully chosen beverages, this cookbook prioritizes nutrition without compromising on flavor or variety. Portion control and meal planning guidance aim to empower seniors with CKD Stage 4 to make informed dietary choices, ensuring balanced nourishment while maintaining kidney health.

The significance of adopting and adapting to this diet cannot be overstated. By following these guidelines and preparing meals from this cookbook, seniors can actively contribute to managing their health, potentially delaying kidney function decline and preventing complications associated with CKD Stage 4. A diet tailored to their needs promotes overall well-being, potentially reducing the risk of cardiovascular issues, bone disorders, and electrolyte imbalances.

For those navigating CKD Stage 4, adopting this diet isn't just about recipes; it's a commitment to enhanced health, improved symptom management, and a better quality of life. The special motivation to embrace this dietary approach lies in the transformative impact it can have on one's health journey. By embracing these culinary offerings and nutritional insights, seniors can take charge of their health, savor delicious meals, and thrive while managing chronic kidney disease.

Remember, every meal prepared from this cookbook isn't just a dish; it's a step towards a healthier and more vibrant life. Embrace this diet, adapt it to your preferences, and witness the profound positive changes it can bring to your health and well-being. Your commitment to this kidney-friendly diet paves the way for a healthier, more fulfilling life even while managing CKD Stage 4.

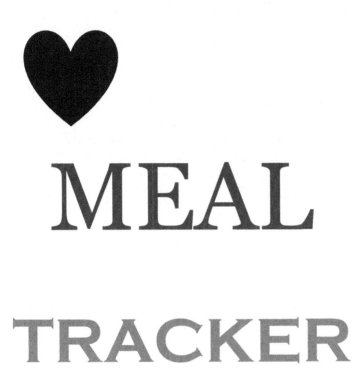

# MEAL

# TRACKER

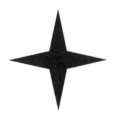

| Monday | Breakfast | Lunch | Dinner |
|--------|-----------|-------|--------|
| | | | |

| Tuesday | Breakfast | Lunch | Dinner |
|---------|-----------|-------|--------|
| | | | |

| Wednesday | Breakfast | Lunch | Dinner |
|-----------|-----------|-------|--------|
| | | | |

| Thursday | Breakfast | Lunch | Dinner |
|----------|-----------|-------|--------|
| | | | |

| Friday | Breakfast | Lunch | Dinner |
|--------|-----------|-------|--------|
| | | | |

| Saturday | Breakfast | Lunch | Dinner |
|----------|-----------|-------|--------|
| | | | |

| Sunday | Breakfast | Lunch | Dinner |
|--------|-----------|-------|--------|
| | | | |

| Monday | Breakfast | Lunch | Dinner |
|---|---|---|---|
| | | | |

| Tuesday | Breakfast | Lunch | Dinner |
|---|---|---|---|
| | | | |

| Wednesday | Breakfast | Lunch | Dinner |
|---|---|---|---|
| | | | |

| Thursday | Breakfast | Lunch | Dinner |
|---|---|---|---|
| | | | |

| Friday | Breakfast | Lunch | Dinner |
|---|---|---|---|
| | | | |

| Saturday | Breakfast | Lunch | Dinner |
|---|---|---|---|
| | | | |

| Sunday | Breakfast | Lunch | Dinner |
|---|---|---|---|
| | | | |

| Monday | Breakfast | Lunch | Dinner |
|---|---|---|---|
| | | | |

| Tuesday | Breakfast | Lunch | Dinner |
|---|---|---|---|
| | | | |

| Wednesday | Breakfast | Lunch | Dinner |
|---|---|---|---|
| | | | |

| Thursday | Breakfast | Lunch | Dinner |
|---|---|---|---|
| | | | |

| Friday | Breakfast | Lunch | Dinner |
|---|---|---|---|
| | | | |

| Saturday | Breakfast | Lunch | Dinner |
|---|---|---|---|
| | | | |

| Sunday | Breakfast | Lunch | Dinner |
|---|---|---|---|
| | | | |

| | Breakfast | Lunch | Dinner |
|---|---|---|---|
| Monday | | | |

| | Breakfast | Lunch | Dinner |
|---|---|---|---|
| Tuesday | | | |

| | Breakfast | Lunch | Dinner |
|---|---|---|---|
| Wednesday | | | |

| | Breakfast | Lunch | Dinner |
|---|---|---|---|
| Thursday | | | |

| | Breakfast | Lunch | Dinner |
|---|---|---|---|
| Friday | | | |

| | Breakfast | Lunch | Dinner |
|---|---|---|---|
| Saturday | | | |

| | Breakfast | Lunch | Dinner |
|---|---|---|---|
| Sunday | | | |

|  | Breakfast | Lunch | Dinner |
|---|---|---|---|
| **Monday** | | | |

|  | Breakfast | Lunch | Dinner |
|---|---|---|---|
| **Tuesday** | | | |

|  | Breakfast | Lunch | Dinner |
|---|---|---|---|
| **Wednesday** | | | |

|  | Breakfast | Lunch | Dinner |
|---|---|---|---|
| **Thursday** | | | |

|  | Breakfast | Lunch | Dinner |
|---|---|---|---|
| **Friday** | | | |

|  | Breakfast | Lunch | Dinner |
|---|---|---|---|
| **Saturday** | | | |

|  | Breakfast | Lunch | Dinner |
|---|---|---|---|
| **Sunday** | | | |

|  | Breakfast | Lunch | Dinner |
|---|---|---|---|
| **Monday** | | | |

|  | Breakfast | Lunch | Dinner |
|---|---|---|---|
| **Tuesday** | | | |

|  | Breakfast | Lunch | Dinner |
|---|---|---|---|
| **Wednesday** | | | |

|  | Breakfast | Lunch | Dinner |
|---|---|---|---|
| **Thursday** | | | |

|  | Breakfast | Lunch | Dinner |
|---|---|---|---|
| **Friday** | | | |

|  | Breakfast | Lunch | Dinner |
|---|---|---|---|
| **Saturday** | | | |

|  | Breakfast | Lunch | Dinner |
|---|---|---|---|
| **Sunday** | | | |

| | Breakfast | Lunch | Dinner |
|---|---|---|---|
| **Monday** | | | |

| | Breakfast | Lunch | Dinner |
|---|---|---|---|
| **Tuesday** | | | |

| | Breakfast | Lunch | Dinner |
|---|---|---|---|
| **Wednesday** | | | |

| | Breakfast | Lunch | Dinner |
|---|---|---|---|
| **Thursday** | | | |

| | Breakfast | Lunch | Dinner |
|---|---|---|---|
| **Friday** | | | |

| | Breakfast | Lunch | Dinner |
|---|---|---|---|
| **Saturday** | | | |

| | Breakfast | Lunch | Dinner |
|---|---|---|---|
| **Sunday** | | | |

| Monday | Breakfast | Lunch | Dinner |
|---|---|---|---|
| | | | |

| Tuesday | Breakfast | Lunch | Dinner |
|---|---|---|---|
| | | | |

| Wednesday | Breakfast | Lunch | Dinner |
|---|---|---|---|
| | | | |

| Thursday | Breakfast | Lunch | Dinner |
|---|---|---|---|
| | | | |

| Friday | Breakfast | Lunch | Dinner |
|---|---|---|---|
| | | | |

| Saturday | Breakfast | Lunch | Dinner |
|---|---|---|---|
| | | | |

| Sunday | Breakfast | Lunch | Dinner |
|---|---|---|---|
| | | | |

| Monday | Breakfast | Lunch | Dinner |
|---|---|---|---|
| | | | |

| Tuesday | Breakfast | Lunch | Dinner |
|---|---|---|---|
| | | | |

| Wednesday | Breakfast | Lunch | Dinner |
|---|---|---|---|
| | | | |

| Thursday | Breakfast | Lunch | Dinner |
|---|---|---|---|
| | | | |

| Friday | Breakfast | Lunch | Dinner |
|---|---|---|---|
| | | | |

| Saturday | Breakfast | Lunch | Dinner |
|---|---|---|---|
| | | | |

| Sunday | Breakfast | Lunch | Dinner |
|---|---|---|---|
| | | | |

| | Breakfast | Lunch | Dinner |
|---|---|---|---|
| Monday | | | |

| | Breakfast | Lunch | Dinner |
|---|---|---|---|
| Tuesday | | | |

| | Breakfast | Lunch | Dinner |
|---|---|---|---|
| Wednesday | | | |

| | Breakfast | Lunch | Dinner |
|---|---|---|---|
| Thursday | | | |

| | Breakfast | Lunch | Dinner |
|---|---|---|---|
| Friday | | | |

| | Breakfast | Lunch | Dinner |
|---|---|---|---|
| Saturday | | | |

| | Breakfast | Lunch | Dinner |
|---|---|---|---|
| Sunday | | | |

Made in United States
North Haven, CT
24 December 2024

63374640R00055